I'm Really Scared....What Can I Do?

A Workbook For Children Experiencing Anxiety, Fears, Panic, Phobias, and Obsessive Compulsive Disorder

By

David E. Miller, Ph.D.

Psychologist

Illustrations By Erin Barker

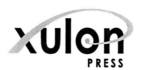

PRESS

I'm Really Scared...What Can I Do?
by David E. Miller, Ph.D.

Printed in the United States of America

ISBN 9781619968783

www.xulnpress.com

Dedication

This book is dedicated to several people who played significant roles in motivating and encouraging me to produce it. Perhaps the most important persons demonstrating the necessity of such a work are the hundreds, perhaps thousands of children that have been a part of my patient roster over the last 25+ years of practice. Through no fault of their own, they were forced to struggle with the discomfort and at times debilitating emotions of fear and anxiety or panic. While some children are reared in families with a family history characteristic of anxiety and seem to learn such a response to stress from the adults in their lives, others sustained trauma that resulted in overwhelming fear, anxiety, panic, or phobic reactions. Some children even develop an extreme form of anxiety known as Obsessive Compulsive Disorder that is characterized by uncontrollable thoughts that seem to present repetitively with little if anything to control or eliminate the thoughts from the child's mind.

Childhood should be exempt from trauma, stress, or significant problems that can stifle normal development; however, we cannot isolate our children or grandchildren exclusively from the forces that can threaten adverse outcomes. Try as we should, their exposure to threats and evil forces that lurk among us are a reality. We as parents and grandparents must carefully guard them and attempt to prevent such forces from adversely affecting their development. However, should our child develop such a reaction as fear, panic, anxiety, a phobia, or even OCD, parents and grandparents need resources that can help these precious little ones overcome the emotions that may circumvent the happiness that should characterize normal childhood. This workbook has been designed as such a resource.

Graphic designer & artist, Erin Barker, deserves special mention for the illustrations provided as coloring pages for the children using this workbook.

Many thanks are due my godly parents, Rev. L.B. and Ruth Miller; their example of the values they wished for me to learn concerning the sanctity of life itself, the joys and happiness that should characterize childhood, and practical ways to address normal fears and anxiety of childhood, was very instrumental in what I have come to believe as important values I thus promote in both my personal and professional life. Consistent support of this work comes from our own children—Scott Alan Miller and his wife, Cara, and Lori Ann (Miller) Hicks, and her husband, Adam. Four precious grandchildren, Kate Elizabeth Miller, Anna Marie Miller, Camden Thaddeus Hicks, and Jagger Cole Hicks, have made the production of this work a high priority as they face the stressors in this life that can threaten fears or anxiety that disrupt happiness in normal childhood. My wife, Joy who consistently upholds me and my patients in prayer, deserves much recognition for her efforts. Her constant encouragement, understanding, and support of my ministry to hurting children and their families, provides much energy and motivation. In many ways, her love and support of my work has enabled me to persevere at times when choosing a more enjoyable hobby would be preferable. Her tender and loving, prayerful support of our grandchildren is most inspiring to me as we attempt to be a supportive resource in their development.

Table of Contents

Child's Handbook Section

Parent's Section of Handbook
With further information

Parent's Notations From Teachers,
Counselors, and their Child's Doctor

Chapter 1

Hey there partner! What you doing? Are you having a good day or a not so good day? Are you having a BAD day?

Oh, I almost forgot...I should introduce myself to you. My name is Tony. I am the oldest kid in my family; I have a younger sister and a younger brother. That makes me the "older brother" that my parents remind me of most of the time.

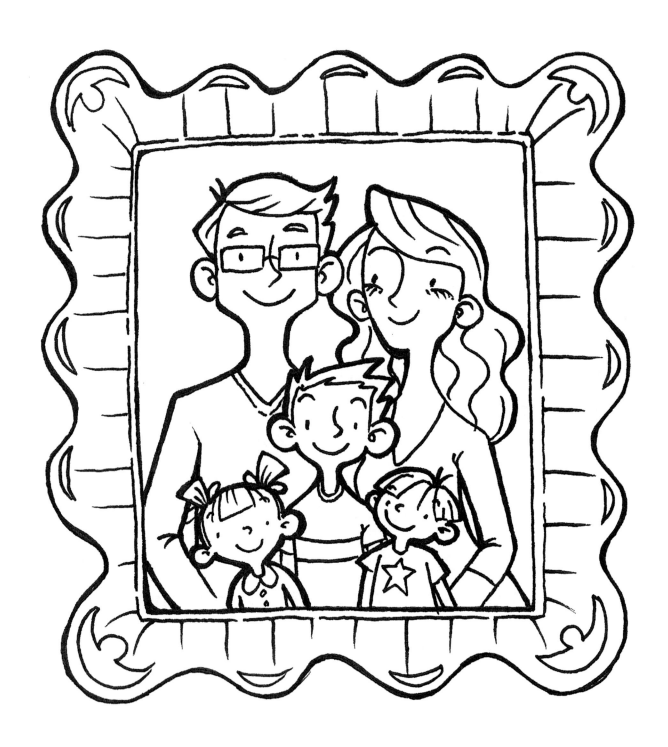

We also have a pet dog—her name is FLUFFY; sometimes we call her FLUFF BALL. She got her name because she is fluffy white and looks very fluffy—almost like a bundle of cotton.

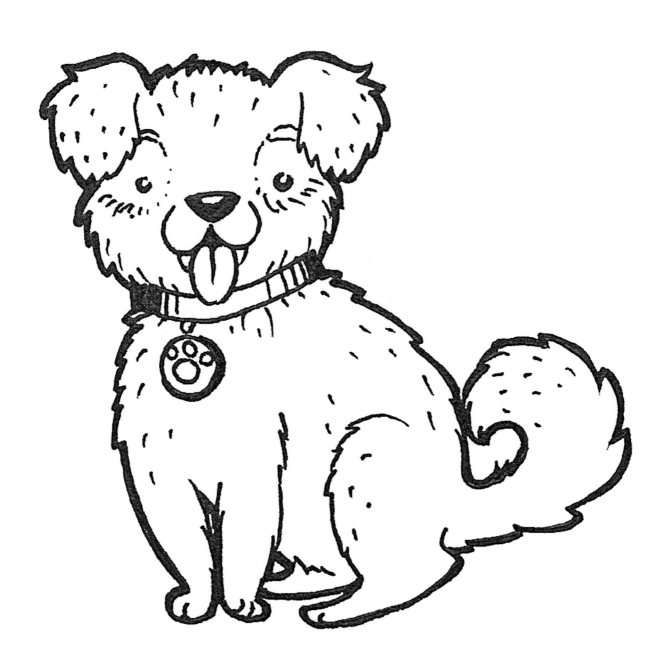

My parents say I have to be an example since my younger sister and brother look up to me and want to be just like me. My parents said it is important that I obey the rules and make good choices since the little guys in my family will likely copy me or follow my example.

I get it...Modeling for my younger sis and bro is important...but not always fun!

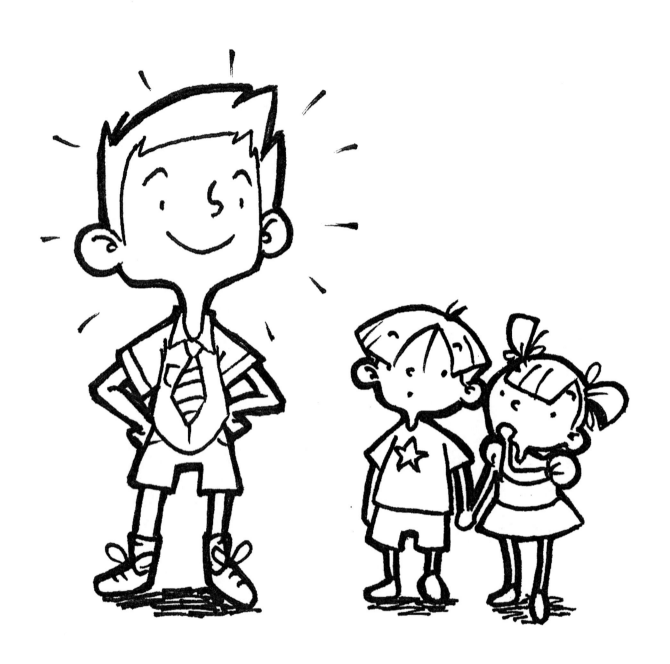

I'm really not sure about all of that—it's kinda hard to think my little sister and brother would want to be like me. You see I have plenty of bad days and I hope they don't catch what I have. I will just call it the "BAD DAY" disease. I wouldn't wish that problem on anyone—it is just awful and I hate being this way. When I'm having one of those days when something goes wrong, I feel very weak and not very proud of myself. I really wish I could be stronger and not have such days.

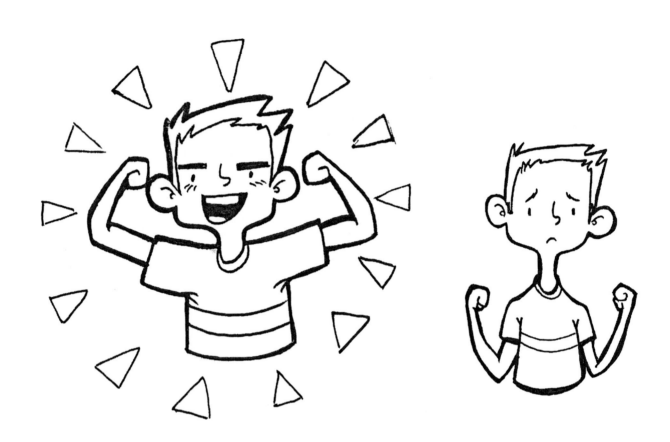

Not all my days are BAD DAYS... some days would actually be GOOD DAYS. On the GOOD DAYS, I am happy and not worried about anything. But I hate the BAD days! They are terrible...and I would do anything to AVOID having one of those days.

Good Days....are good!
Bad Days are Awful!

You ask what is the difference between a GOOD day and a BAD day? I'm really glad you asked! Since you asked me, I will tell you the answer.

A GOOD day is what I would say is a NORMAL day—you know, when things are all going OK; the sun is shining and you can play outside, your friends treat you nicely, you don't seem to do anything to get your parents or the teacher upset with you...you get a good grade on your homework and the teacher compliments you for being a good student...everything just seems to be PERFECT...and you are HAPPY without any worries or problems to deal with.

DON'T YOU JUST WISH EVERYDAY COULD BE A GOOD DAY? I sure do! Life would be so easy, if all my days were GOOD ONES!

I WOULD LOVE IT IF ALL MY DAYS COULD BE

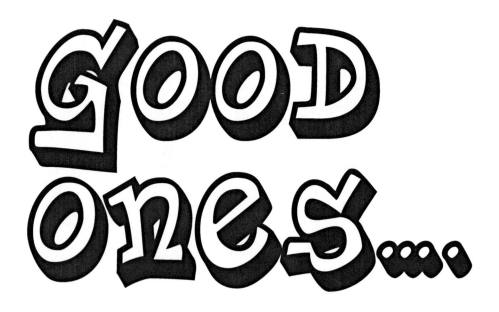

GOOD ONES....

I hate BAD DAYS.

BUT......all days are not good ones and sometimes you have a BAD DAY. Someone famous once said that EVERYONE HAS A BAD DAY

ONCE IN A WHILE and NO ONE HAS ALL GOOD DAYS.

Well, I guess I should tell you what a BAD DAY is...Right? O.K. then, I'll try to tell you what a BAD DAY LOOKS LIKE. A BAD DAY is sort of the opposite of a GOOD DAY. It might mean that even though you planned to play outside with your friends, when you get up on Saturday Morning, you look outside and it is storming and raining really hard; and, of course your mom tells you playing outside today in the storm just isn't an option and you will have to choose some other activity. BOY IS THAT DISAPPOINTING...all my best laid out plans just went down the toilet.

Or a BAD DAY might be when you forgot your homework and both your parents and the teacher get on your case. BOY THAT IS EMBARRASSING—especially when it is in front of the other students. A BAD DAY could be any day where things just don't go the way you expected them to go...and so you feel disappointed or upset.

Even with such disappointments, you can usually get over them pretty easily and find something to do to feel better about things.

Chapter 2

There are REALLY, REALLY BAD days that bring more than just disappointment that you can get over quickly. The REAL BAD DAYS are really hard to understand... they are really scary and make me really, really worried.

My parents got so worried about my BAD DAYS that they took me to see a special doctor called a psychologist. This doctor wasn't like my other doctor that my mom takes me to when I am sick or the one that gives me those shots that all kids have to have as they grow up. This special doctor has helped me learn a lot about BAD DAYS, what causes them...and MOST OF

ALL how to deal with them so I can feel better.

A REALLY BAD DAY can be a day when I feel really scared about something—a FEELING my doctor calls ANXIETY. I asked him what anxiety is, and he said it was simply a feeling of being really, really scared about something. He said I might be scared that something might happen to me or my parents, that I might get lost, or someone would kidnap me. He also said some kids have this "anxiety" after having a bad dream or nightmare. He actually says that nightmares are really common for boys my age and that as I get older, the nightmares sort of go away on their own—not to worry about them. BOY WAS THAT A RELIEF....just to talk with my doctor seems to help me feel better when he tells me that these feelings and experiences are normal and not to worry.

I JUST LOVE IT WHEN MY DOCTOR SAYS..."THIS IS NORMAL" and "NOT TO WORRY!" Of course my parents told me that too, but it seems more important when my doctor tells me. He has studied this sort of thing and has treated many little boys and girls like me...SO I THINK HE KNOWS WHAT HE IS TALKING ABOUT and I'm GOING TO BELIEVE HIM. I told my parents that they were right...according to my doctor and I was glad the doctor agreed with them.

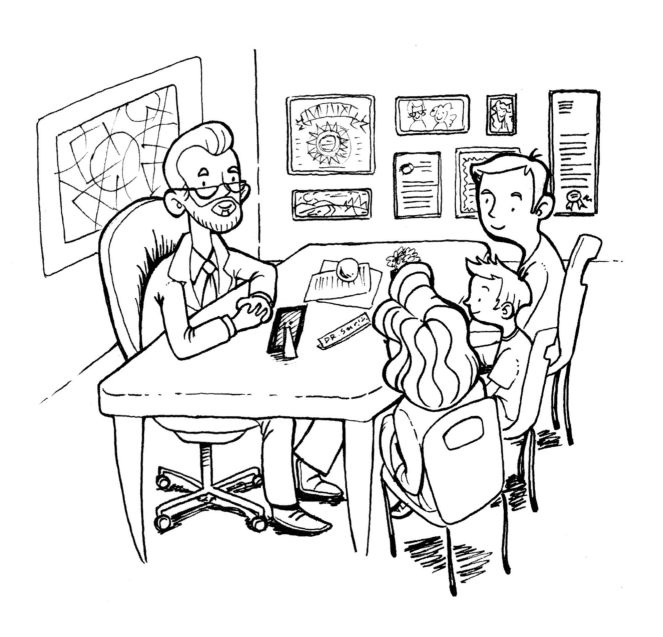

Chapter 3

Another VERY IMPORTANT thing that I learned from my doctor was that many, many people suffer from anxiety or fears. That really made me feel better since at times I felt like I was the only kid who felt this way. My doctor said that actually there are a whole lot of people and kids who struggle with anxiety. THE GOOD NEWS is—they can be helped!

My doctor told me about several different kinds of anxiety. At first, it scared me—I was thinking that I might get all of them and I was having enough trouble with the one I called

BAD DAY DISEASE. But he said not to worry...most of the time people don't get all of them.

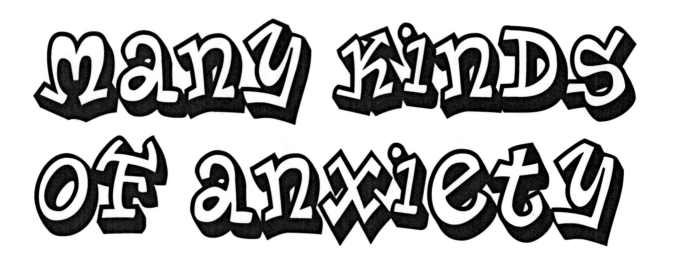

MANY KINDS OF ANXIETY

If you would like, I think I can maybe explain the different kinds to you. My doctor says that the more I know about something...the less scary it seems. So by learning more about things, it makes that thing less scary to us!

GENERAL ANXIETY DISORDER or GAD

The first kind of ANXIETY is just plain GENERAL ANXIETY DISORDER or GAD...it is simply feeling a little scared or having fear most of the time. People with this kind of anxiety worry most of the time about little things—such as having a bad dream, not knowing the answer when the teacher calls on you, forgetting a rule and getting into trouble with the teacher or parents. These things aren't happening, but the person with general anxiety worries it might happen.

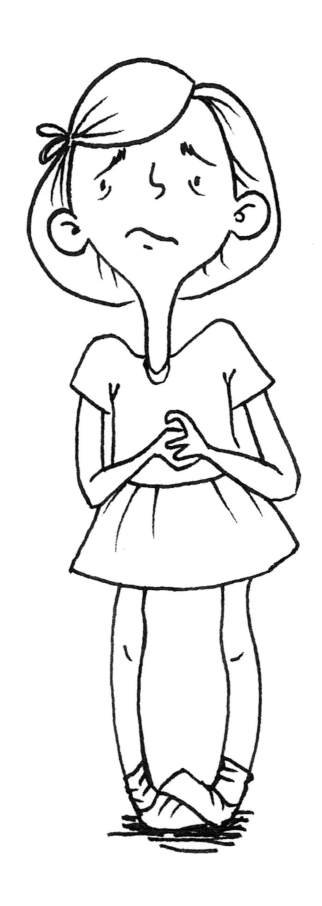

PANIC or PANIC ATTACK

The second kind of anxiety is called Panic or Panic Attack. This form of anxiety is more serious than general anxiety. People who have panic attacks can feel like they are having a heart attack since their hearts beat real fast. They might have a hard time breathing or catching their breath. They may get dizzy, sweaty, and feel weak or like they are going to faint. When they feel these things, they get even more anxious about what is happening to them...they feel helpless since they can't seem to control it or stop it. Sometimes they even call 911 because they think they are having a heart attack or dying.

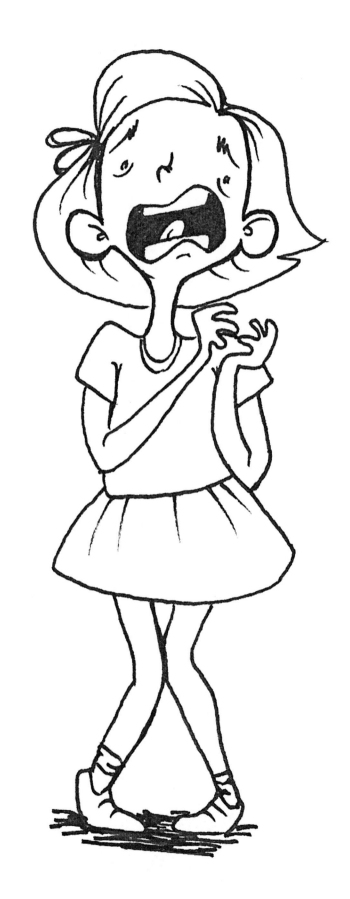

PHOBIA ... PHOBIAS

A Phobia is a rather interesting type of anxiety—it is like you become anxious at one special thing but other things don't make you anxious. My doctor told me that a phobia is sometimes being scared of something that really doesn't pose any threat or risk, yet you feel very anxious about it and fear it. He said sometimes kids have what is called SCHOOL PHOBIA, which is exactly what you are thinking—those kids are scared of school. When he told me this, I thought some days I might have school phobia since I would rather stay home and play computer games...well, I guess not,

I'm really not scared of school; I just find it inconvenient some days when I wish I could do other things. My doctor said that other people develop phobias about going out in public—this is called SOCIAL PHOBIA. Other people have specific fears with things like riding an elevator, climbing a ladder, going down to their basement, flying on an airplane, going through tunnels, riding on escalators or in elevators, certain animals such as dogs or cats, being in too small of a room, and many other things. There are special words for each of these phobias, but I can't say them or spell them so we will just skip over those special words. Basically, my doctor said that people can develop an extreme fear or anxiety for just about anything. He said these things usually are not dangerous and that makes their fear IRRATIONAL or IT DOESN'T MAKE SENSE! However, he said the fear is REAL and it causes EXTREME ANXIETY and people can't seem to get over it on their own. I guess they sort of feel POWERLESS and WEAK.

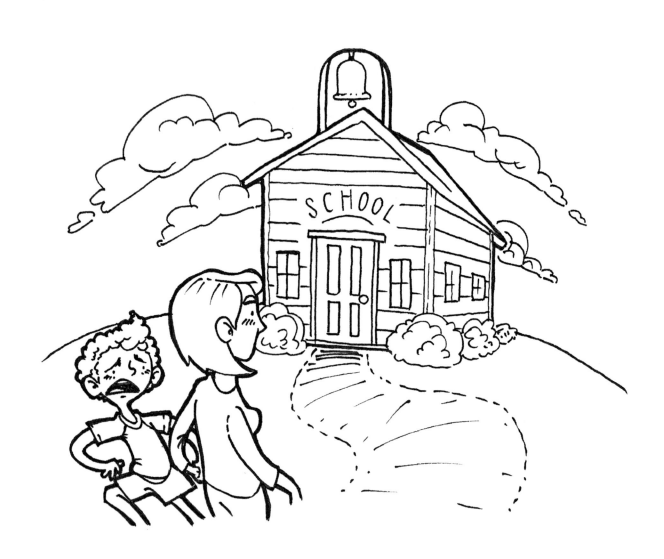

My doctor also told me that some children have nightmares that are called night terrors; I guess those things are REALLY, REALLY BAD nightmares that leave you REALLY, REALLY scared. He said some kids even experience "sleepwalking" during night terrors. I told him that one was hard to understand, but I'd take his word at it. He said the boy or girl is sleeping so soundly and dreaming that they actually get up and walk around the house without even knowing it. I told him that sounded weird; he said he agreed with me and that it seemed weird to the parents as well. I was greatly relieved to hear him say those magical words again…that such things were all considered NORMAL and that these kids also would likely grow out of these bad experiences and not keep having them when they grew up.

NORMAL... MANY THINGS ARE JUST NORMAL!

POST TRAUMATIC STRESS DISORDER

POST TRAUMATIC STRESS DISORDER is a very severe form of anxiety according to my doctor. He said that if something VERY, VERY SCARY happens to a person they can develop this anxiety—he called it PSTD for short. This is the kind of anxiety that some of our soldiers that fought in a war get since they see so many very bad things. PTSD can result after a very scary event that involved physical harm or threat of physical harm such as being in a war, an auto or some other kind of accident, a house fire, a bank when it was being robbed, a plane crash, earthquake or tornado, train wreck, or being kidnapped. These are very scary events and after one happens to you...I guess you really fear that it could happen again and that's what causes the extreme fear called PTSD.

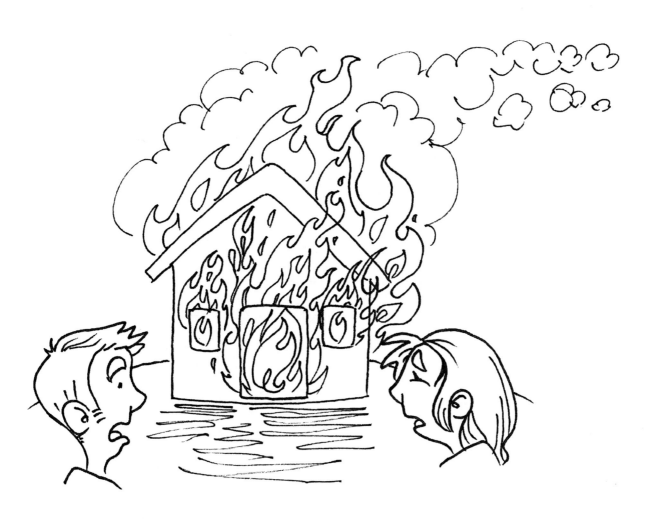

OBSESSIVE-COMPULSIVE DISORDER

OBSESSIVE-COMPULSIVE DISORDER or OCD for short is a specialized anxiety. People who have OCD have unwanted thoughts that they can't seem to get out of their minds. These thoughts just keep coming and coming no matter what they try to do. The thoughts can involve fears or worries such as something bad happening to them or their families, that they forgot to do something like turn the stove off or lock their door, washing their hands many times because of possible germs, and other such things. My doctor said that people with OCD usually begin doing things, called compulsions, to help get the thought out of their mind. He said that the thought is called an OBSESSION and the act the person does to get rid of the thought is called COMPULSION. He gave me an example of the person who feared he had germs on his hands will begin washing his hands many times a day—even causing his skin to get too dry and sometimes cause breaks in the skin that require ointment. While washing your hands is important to do after you go to the bathroom or play outside in the dirt, he said these people wash their hands 30-40 or more times a day and this is extreme and not necessary. He also said that some people with OCD will develop other habits like needing to count things, touch things as they go by them such as poles on a fence, they might collect things and can't get rid of trash, others try to be perfect and keep starting their homework papers over and over again rather than erasing their answer and correcting it. Some people even develop certain ways of doing something and they always do it the very same way—I guess this is what my doctor called a ritual.

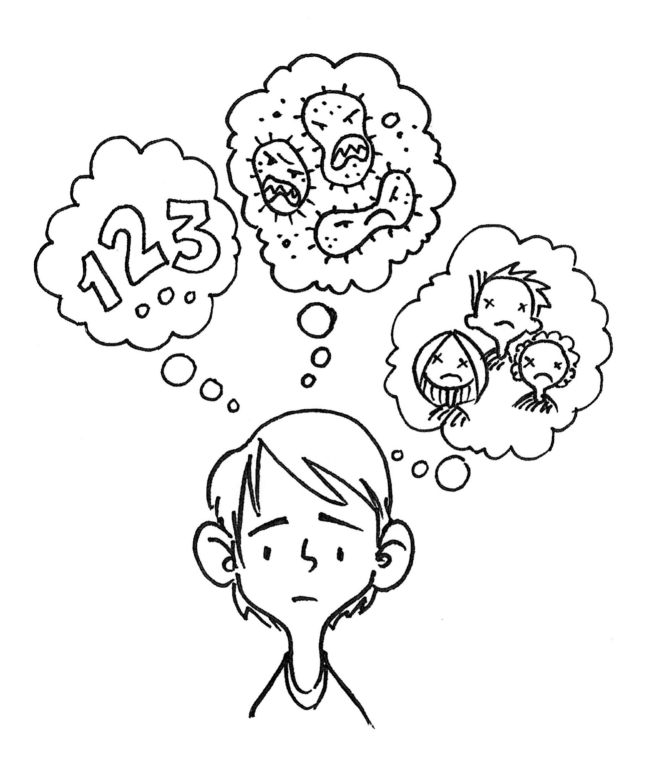

I told my doctor that this form of anxiety seemed really weird and very serious. He agreed with me and said it was one of the more serious types of anxiety—but he said it could be treated and these people can really get better. WOW, that was a relief for me! I told him I didn't think I had this kind of anxiety, but it was really nice to hear that they can get better just like the people who have the less serious kinds.

Chapter 4

Well, now that you know the different kinds of anxiety...would you like to hear what me and my doctor discussed about how to deal with them? I'm sure you do, so I will share everything he told me. If you are a kid with this kind of problem—I want you to get the same help I was given so you can better control it.

You will remember that I told you that my family and I had a pet dog named FLUFFY or FLUFF BALL. We were able to teach Fluffy several tricks like "Sitting," "Laying Down," "Speaking," and even keeping a balloon up in the air like a seal does in a circus show. Fluffy likes to perform these tricks for our guests and of course they really think she is a smart dog and it makes them laugh. I think Fluffy thinks that any visitor we have at my home is coming to see her; and so she puts on her little show for them. Sometimes we have to correct her and make her settle down if she starts racing around our furniture as if she is running a marathon race.

My doctor told me that if my dog Fluffy, who has a rather small brain compared to mine, could learn tricks, I should be able to learn a whole lot more tricks since my brain was more powerful than hers. He said learning how to manage anxiety is sort of like learning tricks—

usually called COPING SKILLS.
My doctor said the more coping
skills or tricks that I have to use,
the BETTER I CAN CONTROL MY
ANXIETY.

COPING SKILLS ARE REALLY JUST TRICKS

My doctor asked me if I wanted to learn some of those tricks. I said, "I'm really glad you asked me...I don't want to learn just some, I want to learn as many as I can learn." My doctor smiled. I think my doctor likes me. He probably thinks I'm a good patient and doctors tend to like patients like me that are cooperative and want to get better.

My doctor said, "Then let's make a list of the tricks you can learn to help you handle anxiety." So here goes...

MY LIST OF TRICKS OR COPING SKILLS

1. RECOGNIZE IT: When I am getting anxious, I simply recognize it, admit it, and then I can deal with it! My doctor said some people keep being anxious since they don't want to admit it—he calls that DENIAL. My doctor said if I am getting scared or anxious, I should just stop and tell myself right then and

there, "Wow...this is making me a little anxious or scared!" I'm not sure why it is, but my doctor said that when you just do this—it seems to give you more control over your anxiety. I guess you are more willing to let someone else know when you admit it to yourself. Recognizing it and admitting it leads to the second trick—Talking about it!

2. TALKING ABOUT It will help since when TALKING ABOUT IT, you usually get MORE INFORMATION which will become our third trick in the list. My doctor said it is important in dealing with any problem, that you recognize it...then be willing to share it with someone you trust. He

said that fears or anxiety can build up inside of someone just like air causes a balloon to get bigger and bigger as more air is blown into it. I guess if we don't talk with anyone about our fears, they build up and seem worse the more we wait to say anything. When we talk about them, it is sort of like letting some of the air out of the balloon. The balloon gets smaller and has less pressure in it; my doctor says that when we talk about our fears with someone, some of the pressure is released and we feel a little better since we "have less pressure" inside of us.

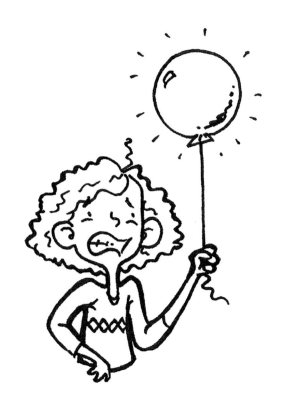

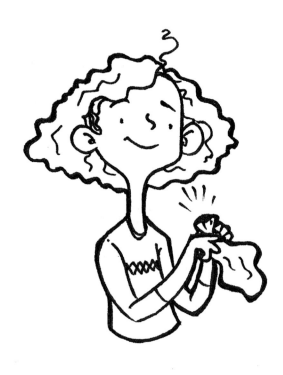

3. The third trick my doctor explained is GETTING MORE KNOWLEDGE about the thing that causes you to be scared or afraid. My doctor said that

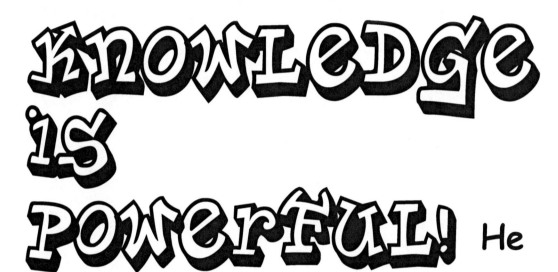 He

said most of the things that scare us are things we know little about. As we learn more about these things, we are less scared. SO...SHARING YOUR FEARS with parents or other people in your life is important. They can help you learn more about these things which should reduce the fear or anxiety you have about that thing. I remember when I started Pre-School that I was really scared. My mom decided to make a special trip to the pre-school so I could look around and get to know where things were. As I became more familiar with the pre-school, I wasn't so scared. So on my first day of school, I had already been there and so it wasn't so new and scary for me. A Pre-Visit to a new school really helped settle my fears.

My doctor told me that he once treated a little girl who was very scared of snakes. That was a real problem for her since her family was missionaries to Africa where there are lots of snakes all over the land. She was struggling so badly that they had to come back home for a while so she could get the help she needed. My doctor had her do a research project on snakes. You might ask why he was acting like her teacher rather than her doctor. He said he wanted her to LEARN MORE about snakes. Of course that wasn't the only thing they did in her treatment, but my doctor said this was an important part of it. The more she learned about snakes, the less fearful she became. She got better... and they returned to Africa to remain as missionaries. SO I GUESS THIS TRICK—Talking about it...and getting more knowledge is an important trick! I'm going to remember this one—it's very simple to do; I'll just pretend I have a report to do for my teacher at school and do my research on whatever scares me.

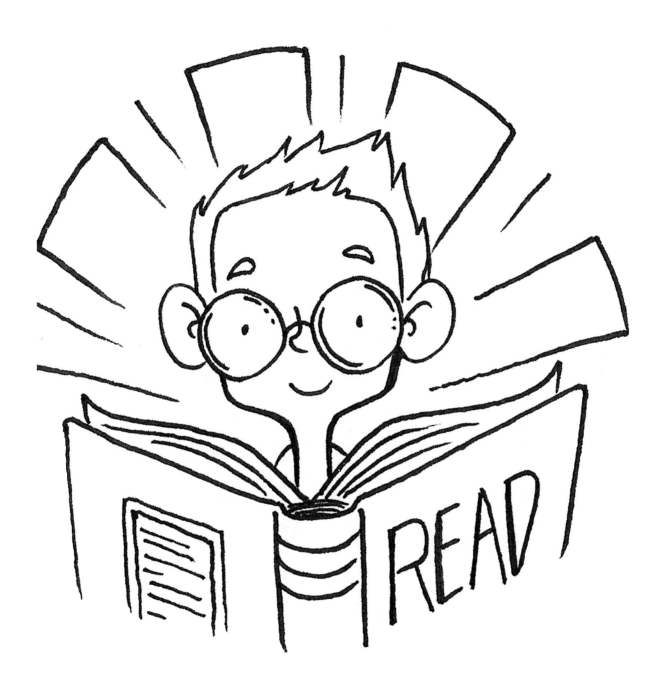

4. My doctor explained the next trick as something he called SELF-TALK or ST for short and LOGICAL PROBLEM SOLVING or LPS for short. He said that self-talk did not mean actually walking around talking to yourself out loud; that would probably seem pretty weird and cause people to think you might be crazy. My doctor said it is sort of like talking to yourself in your mind—thinking things through. He even gave me two questions to ask myself during these self talk sessions. The 2 questions he suggested I ask myself are:

   1. Is this FEAR real or just imagined?

2. Is there something causing this fear or anxiety or is it just a feeling without any evidence?

My doctor said that many fears are merely feelings without any evidence or cause. If I am having fear like there is a hungry lion after me and looking straight at me as he is rubbing his tummy, it is only real if in fact I see the lion in front of me and about to grab me for his lunch. If I am just having that feeling but there is no lion——it is false, not true...there is NO EVIDENCE!

Very similar to SELF TALK is LOGICAL PROBLEM SOLVING or LPS for short. Logical problem solving is just like what it sounds—

stopping yourself for a minute, evaluating the situation...then finding an answer to the problem. Let's see if I can explain how my doctor said this one works: if I'm scared of having a bad nightmare since I have been having nightmares for a while, I would problem solve it by asking myself the following questions:

1. What is my problem?
   <u>My answer</u>: having a bad nightmare
2. What do I know about nightmares?
   <u>My answer</u>: they are just dreams and not real; yes they are scary...but not real!
3. Has any of my nightmares ever come true?
   <u>My Answer</u>: NO

4. What has helped me in the past when having a nightmare?
   <u>My Answer</u>: Waking up, telling mom or dad and getting a hug from them, getting a drink, then going back to sleep

5. CONCLUSION: Since I know this about nightmares and have always survived them in the past...I will just use this plan if I have one and THINGS WILL BE OK! I guess I don't have to worry about nightmares...I have a plan!

ALL MY PROBLEMS CAN BE SOLVED...

I JUST need A PLAN!

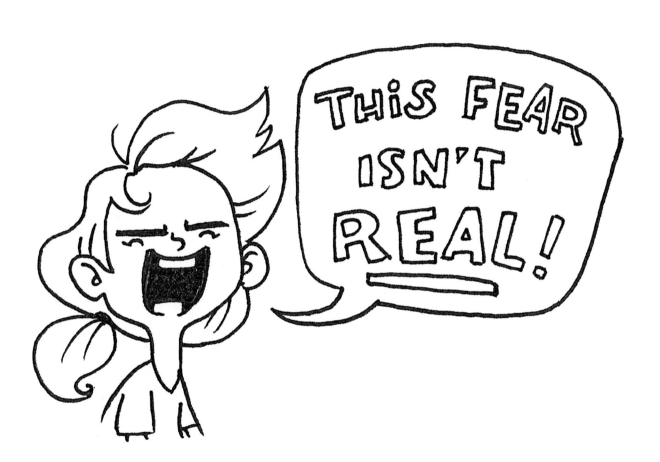

That brings me to the next trick my doctor shared with me—it is called THOUGHT STOPPING!

5. THOUGHT STOPPING or ST for short is exactly what you think it is...it is just

STOPPING the

thought that is causing you to be scared. After you decide there is NO EVIDENCE and the fear is FALSE or NOT TRUE, then you JUST DISMISS IT. Kick it out of your mind! Flush it down the toilet! It's like you tell yourself, "TONY, I know you are having a fear right now, but the feeling isn't true since there is NO EVIDENCE...SO JUST IGNORE IT or DISMISS

IT! SAY GOOD BYE TO THE THOUGHT!

My doctor said it is very important to remember that the fear or anxiety is certainly a REAL THING... but if there is no evidence, it is merely a feeling. At that point, I SHOULD DISMISS IT and say it isn't REAL—it is FALSE. This is what my doctor calls

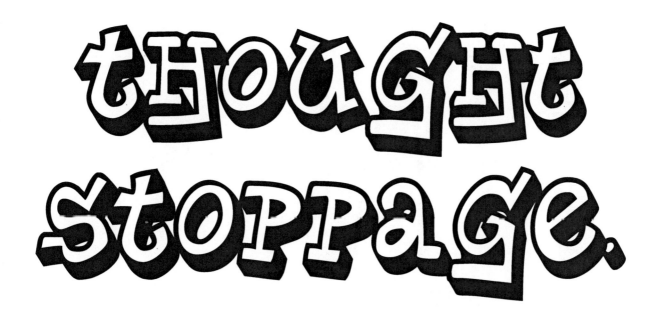

THOUGHT STOPPAGE.

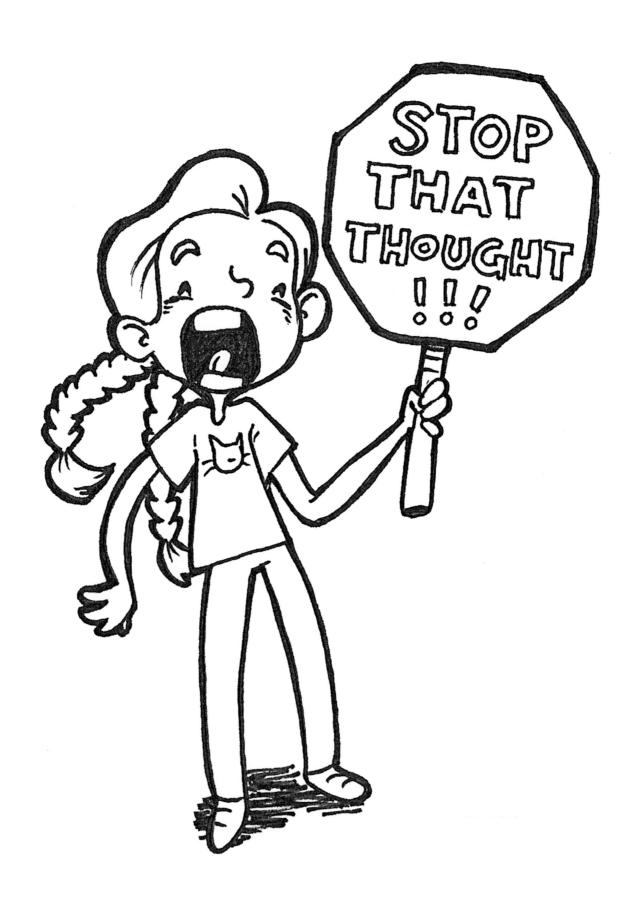

He also said if the thought or fear is like an obsession in OCD, I should try to be very brave and just handle this fear or thought as best as I can for about 15 minutes... since it usually gets weaker and is easier to remove it from your mind then. For example, if I am fearful my hands have germs on them (the thought or obsession) but I have already washed them...I should avoid washing them again (the act or compulsion) for at least 15 minutes...then the feeling (thought or obsession) I need to wash them again will be weaker and probably I can make it go away. That's easy enough...15 minutes isn't that long; I can wait that long, I'm sure!

The 15 Minute rule

He said it is easier to do this trick if you combine it with the next one—RE-FOCUSING ON SOMETHING ELSE!

++++++++++++++++++++++

I want to learn how to Re-focus......

6. RE-FOCUSING ON SOMETHING ELSE means that you get your mind to start thinking about something else. It is harder for your mind to stay focused on the fear or being scared, if you think about something else on

purpose. My doctor said that thinking about something that is fun or a memory that really made me happy are the best things to re-focus on since it is more fun to think about happy things. I asked him to explain further and he said that I could try to remember a fun trip to an amusement park or perhaps a vacation with my family. He said that some kids like to think about the next computer game they wish to buy, or what they want for their birthday coming up, etc. etc. etc.

I guess it would be sort of hard to keep on being scared if you get your mind on something that is fun and exciting.

My doctor said that it is very important that you re-focus your mind on something that is FUN, EXCITING, or ENJOYABLE! I think I can do that...I have lots of exciting things happening to me.

7. EXPOSURE is the seventh trick my doctor shared with me. I guess sometimes this trick is called

DE-SENSITIZATION

since it helps to "de-sensitize" the person to the fear he or she has, but we will just refer to it as exposure or EXP for short. Now this one is an interesting trick...it might be a little harder to understand. My doctor said that if something really is scary like going down to the basement alone, you can take small steps or "baby steps" toward the goal—like the first day, going down 3-4 steps, then the next day going down to maybe 6-7 steps...and progressing a little each day until you get all the way down to the bottom of the stairs. In little steps, you get closer and closer to your goal of being able to go down to the basement. Then you start trying to stay down in the basement for a couple of minutes on the first day you accomplish the goal, then add some minutes the next day... keep adding minutes until you can stay down in the basement for several minutes. He said it is sort of like "exposing" yourself to the thing that makes you fearful...until you conquer it by proving to yourself that YOU CAN DO IT! It like makes you not so sensitive to the thing that you are over sensitive about!

OK, I got it...DECREASING MY SENSITIVITY...How cool is that?

I know that will take lots of courage...anytime you are facing the thing that brings on fear, it is like facing your giant—but it can help you prove to yourself you can conquer the GIANT! This trick is not quick and easy...it takes several days and is in several steps. But my doctor said it is

a good trick and he has used
it with many children as they
conquered their fears.

I can and will conquer the

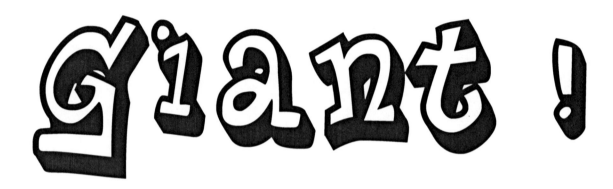

My doctor told me that he once treated a little girl who had become extremely fearful of school buses. He said she had developed a PHOBIA of school buses after an accident. I guess she was getting off the school bus one day and her coat got caught in the door of the school bus and she was dragged for several feet before the bus driver knew she was caught in the door. She was taken to the hospital and treated for some scrapes and scratches on her skin. But the real problem was that she developed so much fear about school buses she couldn't even think about riding one ever again. My doctor knew just what to do...he said he planned to used EXPOSURE with her to help her conquer her fears. He said that one of the first steps in treating her involved having her color pictures of school buses...that was all she could handle as a first step. The next steps progressed to talking about the accident, listening to sounds of school buses, and little by little they made progress until one day my doctor said he arranged for the school bus to come to his office and the little girl, her mother, and my doctor took a short ride in the bus. He said that was really cool since school buses don't ever come to his office to pick up kids going to school. The little girl eventually was able to ride the bus to school if she sat in the back seat and her mother followed the bus in her car. Eventually, the little girl could ride the bus again without her mother following in the car. SHE HAD CONQUERED HER PHOBIA OF

SCHOOL BUSES. She conquered her GIANT—that big, bad, mean yellow box on wheels called a school bus. Now she can ride any school bus and does it every day to and from her school.

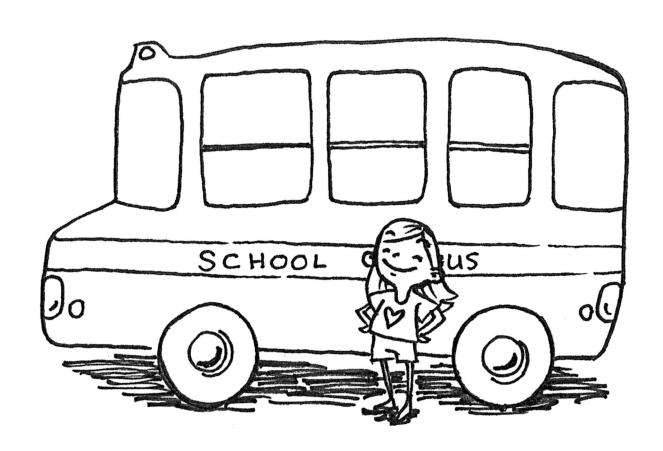

8. The eighth trick that my doctor shared with me is what he called Cognitive-Behavioral Therapy or CBT for short. He said it is a lot like the second trick of TALKING ABOUT IT and is sort of what we were doing as we discussed my problem and discovered ways to help with the problems. He said that our "talking" was the cognitive part and that the "actions" and things we do or practice is the behavioral part. I told him that I liked using CBT since it meant coming to see him and talking about these things. I told him he was REALLY HELPING ME so this CBT must work pretty well! I think he liked that—you know getting a compliment. I think it made him feel good that he was helping me.

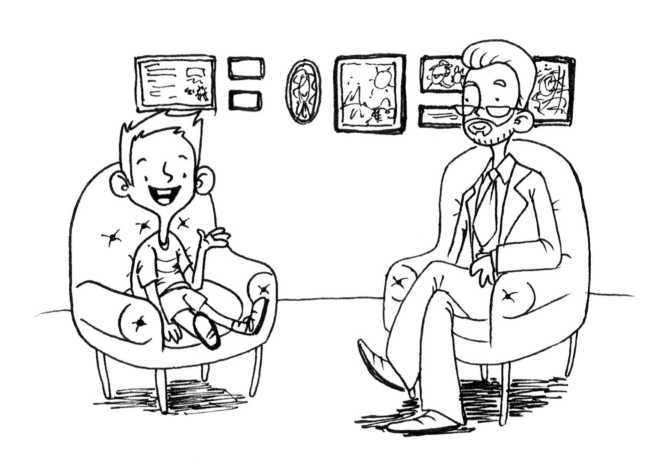

9. According to my doctor, another trick or helpful tool used to help people with anxiety is MEDICINE prescribed by their regular doctor or Pediatrician. My doctor said that sometimes our bodies need medicine to help them work better with "balancing" out the chemicals inside us. He said that sometimes when we experience emotional reactions, our chemical system gets kind of out of balance and the medicine can help to RE-BALANCE things as you work on learning these tricks. My doctor said that medicine is safe and that my regular doctor would know the kind of medicine to prescribe and would watch me closely to make sure it worked and didn't have any harmful effects. He

said that psychologists work real closely with pediatricians when medicine is used as part of the treatment—it is sort of like they are a TEAM and work together to help the boy or girl get better.

He said that some special types of anxiety like OCD or OBSESSIVE COMPULSIVE DISORDER usually only gets better when both medicine and CBT (Cognitive Behavioral Therapy) are used together. I guess that particular type of anxiety doesn't do very well with just medicine or just therapy—but if both are combined, even OCD can get much better. THAT IS GOOD NEWS FOR PEOPLE WHO HAVE OCD!

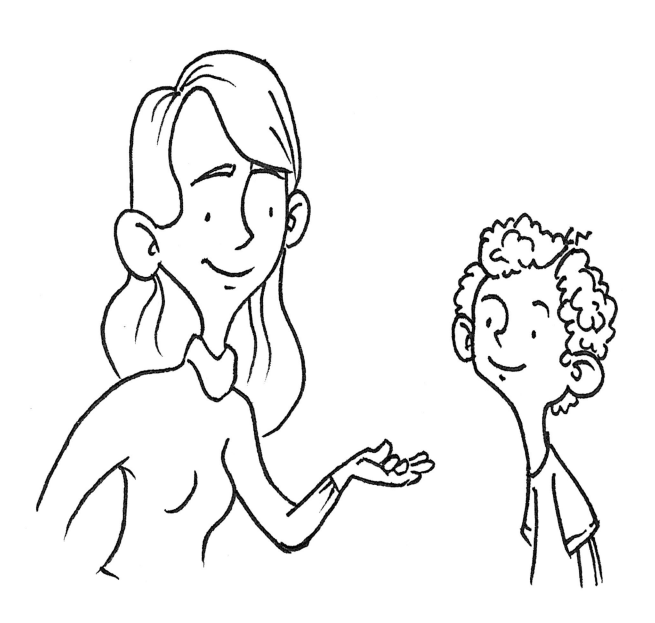

10. My doctor said he doesn't like to refer to this last one as a trick, but rather a helpful tool since it is a spiritual thing and that it involved my religious value system and belief in GOD. He said that since GOD created Adam & Eve in the beginning of time, He knew all about how we work, think, and feel. God actually created our emotions and my doctor said he believed that we were made pretty WONDERFULLY in the image of GOD. He said that God knows when we are scared or anxious, fearful, fretful, or feeling very overwhelmed with worries.

I listened to everything
my doctor was telling me...
finally, I said "OK, I agree
with all that stuff as my
parents and my teacher
in Sunday school tell me
the same thing...WHAT
IS THIS LAST HELPFUL
TOOL if that's what we
are going to call it?" My
doctor said this tool is a
very serious thing and really
an important and essential
habit we should all do daily.
He then asked me if I
had figured out what this
tool was; and, I said "I
think so." I asked, "Is it
to pray?" He said, "YES...
PRAYER is essential and
very helpful when a boy or
girl is trying to get over

anxiety, phobia, panic, fears, or even obsessive-compulsive disorders."

My doctor said that the BIBLE describes times when JESUS experienced fears and anxiety. It was at these times that He prayed to God his Father for help and strength. My doctor said we can follow the example of JESUS and it would help us in overcoming our fears. Just like GOD helped JESUS, He will help us. My doctor said it is important to have FAITH that prayer will be helpful and that GOD cares about us. He said that some important research a few years ago discovered that doctors who pray with their patients find that their patients get better sooner than other patients. Now that is pretty cool! RESEARCH even proves that prayer works!

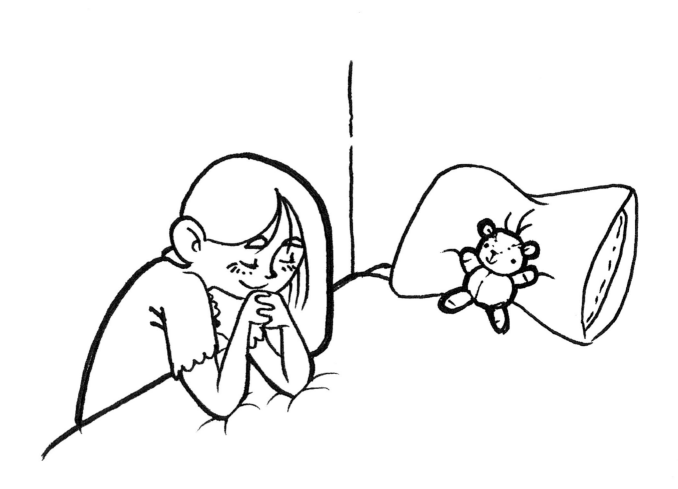

So that's about the end of my story and what I know about good days and bad days...anxiety, fears, being scared, and even such things as phobias, OCD, and panic. I hope these tricks will HELP YOU as they do me. I still have some anxiety from time to time, but I have a PLAN and can usually get over it pretty well.

The END OF MY STORY

FURTHER INFORMATION FOR PARENTS

Characteristics Of Various Forms Of Anxiety
(as specified in Diagnostic and Statistical Manual of Mental Disorders, Fourth Edition, Text Revision, published by American Psychiatric Association, Washington, DC, 2000)

Generalized Anxiety Disorder or GAD

Excessive anxiety and worry (apprehensive expectation), occurring more days than not for at least 6 months, about a number of events or activities (such as work or school performance)

Anxiety and worry are associated with three or more of the following six symptoms (with at least some symptoms present for more days than not for the past 6 months):
  (1) Restlessness or feeling keyed up or on edge
  (2) Being easily fatigued
  (3) Difficulty concentrating or mind going blank
  (4) Irritability
  (5) Muscle tension
  (6) Sleep disturbance (difficulty falling or staying asleep, or restless unsatisfying sleep)
The anxiety, worry, or physical symptoms cause clinically significant distress or impairment in social, occupational, or other important areas of functioning

Panic or Panic Attack

A discrete period of intense fear or discomfort, in which four (or more) of the following symptoms developed abruptly and reached a peak within 10 minutes:
  (1) Palpitations, pounding heart, or accelerated heart rate
  (2) Sweating
  (3) Trembling or shaking
  (4) Sensations of shortness of breath or smothering
  (5) Feeling of choking
  (6) Pain or discomfort
  (7) Nausea or abdominal distress
  (8) Feeling dizzy, unsteady, lightheaded, or faint
  (9) De-realization (feelings of unreality) or depersonalization (being detached from oneself)
  (10)   Fear of losing control or going crazy
  (11)   Fear of dying
  (12)   Paresthesias (numbness or tingling sensations)
  (13)   Chills or hot flushes

Panic Disorder Without Agoraphobia
Experiencing the above features of panic attack, but not finding it difficult to leave home

Panic Disorder With Agoraphobia
Experiencing the above features of panic attack; and, also finding it difficult to leave home or go out in public

Phobia or Phobias
Marked and persistent fear that is excessive or unreasonable, cued by the presence or anticipation of a specific object(s) or situation(s) (i.e. flying, heights, animals, receiving an injection, seeing blood)

Exposure to the phobic stimulus almost invariably provokes an immediate anxiety response, which may take the form of a situational bound or predisposed panic – anxiety in children are often expressed by crying, tantrums, freezing, or clinging

Phobic situations are generally avoided or else is endured with intense anxiety or distress

Specific Types of Phobia(s):
   Animal Type: fear is cued by animals or insects
   Natural Environment Type: fear is cued by objects in the natural environment, such as storms, heights, or water
   Blood-injection -Injury Type: fear is cued by seeing blood or an injury or by receiving an injection or other invasive medical procedures
   Situational Type: fear is cued by a specific situation such as public transportation, tunnels, bridges, elevators, flying, driving, or enclosed places

Specific Sub-Types of Phobia(s):
   (1) Social Phobia (Social Anxiety Disorder): marked and persistent fear of one or more social or performance situations in which the child is exposed to unfamiliar people or to possible scrutiny by others when there is evidence of the capacity for age-appropriate social relationships with familiar people in a peer setting
   (2) School Phobia: same as above with school being the specific setting

Post Traumatic Stress Disorder or PTSD:
Child has been exposed to a traumatic event in which both of the following were present:
   (1) The child experienced, witnessed, or was confronted with an event or events that involved actual or threatened death or serious injury, or a threat to the physical integrity of self or others
   (2) The child's response involved intense fear, helplessness, or horror—in children often expressed by disorganized or agitated behavior

The traumatic event is persistently re-experienced in one or more of the following ways:

(1) Recurrent and intrusive distressing recollections of the event, including images, thoughts, or perceptions—in children, repetitive play may occur in which themes or aspects of the trauma are expressed
(2) Recurrent distressing dreams of the event—in children, there may be frightening dreams without recognizable content
(3) Acting or feeling as if the traumatic event were recurring (includes a sense of reliving the experience, illusions, hallucination, and dissociative flashback episodes, including those that occur on awakening)—in children, trauma-specific reenactment may occur
(4) Intense psychological distress at exposure to internal or external cues that symbolize or resemble an aspect of the traumatic event
(5) Physiological reactivity on exposure to internal or external cues that symbolize or resemble an aspect of the traumatic event

Persistent avoidance of stimuli associated with the trauma and numbing of general responsiveness (not present before the trauma), as indicated by three of more of the following:

(1) Efforts to avoid thoughts, feelings, or conversations associated with the trauma
(2) Efforts to avoid activities, places, or people that arouse recollections of the trauma
(3) Inability to recall an important aspect of the trauma
(4) Markedly diminished interest or participation in significant activities
(5) Feeling of detachment or estrangement from others
(6) Restricted range of affect (i.e. unable to have loving feelings)
(7) Sense of a foreshortened future (i.e. does not expect to have a career, marriage, children, or a normal life span

Obsessive-Compulsive Disorder
Experiencing either obsessions or compulsions or both

Obsessions are:
(1) Recurrent and persistent thoughts, impulses, or images that are experienced, at some time during the disturbance, as intrusive and inappropriate and that cause marked anxiety or distress
(2) These thoughts, impulses, or images are not simply excessive worries about real-life problems

Compulsions are:
(1) Repetitive behaviors (e.g. hand washing, ordering, checking) or mental acts (e.g. praying, counting, repeating words silently) that the child feels driven

to perform in response to an obsession, or according to rules that must be applied rigidly
(2) These behaviors or mental acts are aimed at preventing or reducing distress or preventing some dreaded event or situation; however, these behaviors or mental acts either are not connected in a realistic way with what they are designed to neutralize or prevent or are clearly excessive

Obsessions or compulsions cause marked distress, are time consuming (take more than 1 hour a day), or significantly interfere with the child's normal routine, functioning, or usual social activities and relationships

COMMON OBSESSIONS & COMPULSIONS

TYPICAL OBSESSIONS MAY INCLUDE:
- Fear of harm from germs, contamination, or a toxic substance
- Worry that a burglar may break into the home
- Worry about catching a serious illness or having one and not aware of it
- Fear of harm coming to or losing a parent or loved one
- Fear of something bad happening in association with a particular number
- Fear of misplacing or throwing something away in the trash that is really important
- Fear of thinking evil or sinful thoughts that is contrary to one's religious beliefs
- Fear of committing a sin—perhaps the unpardonable sin
- Extreme concern with order, symmetry, or exactness
- Fear of catching AIDS
- Disgust over body wastes or secretions
- Recurring thoughts or images of a sexual nature
- Fear of committing a crime, such as theft
- Recurring thoughts about harming or killing others or oneself
- Fear that some disaster will occur
- Extreme concern with certain sounds, images, words, or numbers

COMMON COMPULSIONS OR RITUALS MAY INCLUDE:
- Excessive hand washing, showering, cleaning, and doing these behaviors in a rather particular or unique manner or sequence
- Touching certain objects in a specific way
- Checking locks, windows, light switches, temperature repeatedly
- Repeating certain actions, such as going through a doorway
- Checking or asking others for reassurance, requesting doctor visits
- Counting over and over to a certain number
- Slowness, excessive caution, dressing "correctly" and undressing repeatedly, grooming repeatedly
- Hoarding, collecting, sorting or the opposite with excessively purging or removing things from possession to streamline things in possession to bare minimum
- Arranging, ordering, or straightening up in a certain way or manner
- Praying, confessing, asking for reassurance.

TREATMENT OF CHILDREN EXPERIENCING ANXIETY PROBLEMS

Generally, the treatment for children experiencing problems with anxiety must involve several steps in process:

(1) Evaluation to thoroughly diagnose this condition and rule out other factors that may appear to manifest the same symptoms

(2) Environmental alterations to reduce level of stimulation and to significantly increase the level of structure within the child's environment, thus increasing a sense of security and predictability for the child

(3) Assess and insure that expectations on child by parental and authority figures is age appropriate and consistent between care givers

(4) Cognitive-Behavioral therapy to help child develop and learn coping skills or strategies that will enable better management of anxiety and anxiety related symptoms

(5) Cognitive-Behavioral therapy to help child learn that experiencing anxiety is a real medical condition and does not mean that he or she is weak; and, with appropriate treatment and changes in thinking, most people with anxiety problems get better

(6) Cognitive-Behavioral therapy to help child learn that some environmental changes or following certain rules or procedures can help reduce the negative effects of anxiety

(7) Evaluation of symptoms to determine if medication, in conjunction with therapy, might be helpful in management of anxiety symptoms

WHEN MEDICATION IS RECOMMENDED AS PART OF THE CHILD'S TREATMENT

Medication is usually not an initial step in treating children with anxiety problems, but, one that might be considered later in the process. To only medicate a child who is exhibiting symptoms of anxiety will not help in the constructive learning of coping skills and alternative thinking that is necessary to conquer anxiety problems. Both behavioral therapy and environmental interventions, including an increase in structure for the child, will be absolutely necessary even if medication is indicated.

Medication will not cure or eliminate anxiety problems, but it can help keep them under control while the child undergoes therapy to learn new coping skills and ways to better manage anxiety symptoms. Medication must be prescribed by a physician—Pediatrician, Family Physician, or Psychiatrist. The physician will work with the counselor, therapist, or psychologist who is providing therapy for the child and his/her family. A "team" approach with the family, therapist, and physician is most important for maximum success in treatment.

Before taking medication for an anxiety disorder:
·   Ask the physician to tell you about the effects and side effects expected from the medication
·   Be sure to inform the physician about any alternative therapies, herbal products, or over-the-counter medications you are taking for any condition
·   Ask the physician when and how the medication should be taken; how and when to stop taking it as some medications cannot be stopped abruptly, but a slower tapering is more desirable
·   Consult with and work with the physician to determine which medication is the right one for your child
·   Remember that some medications are effective only if they are taken regularly and that symptoms may recur if the medication is stopped or dosage altered

When medication is indicated as part of the treatment approach for a child, extreme care is given in the selection of appropriate medications and then monitored very closely by the child's pediatrician or family physician. Fortunately, over the years, physicians and pediatricians have learned better ways to prescribe the medications and have slowed the whole process down. Rather than starting a child on the therapeutic dosage as recommended by the PDR according to the child's age and weight, the new approach to starting medication is very different. Generally, the beginning dosages of such medications are only $\frac{1}{2}$ the therapeutic dosage or a very small dosage, which we know is not going to be effective in controlling the symptoms.

We start the medication at this ineffective dosage for the first few days so that the child's body can get use to the medication. After the first few days (7—10 days), the medication is moved upward. We call this "titration" which means a gradual increase of the medication to what the appropriate dosage should be. By slowing down the introduction of the medication to the body, we can certainly reduce the side effects the child could experience, and many times eliminate possible side effects all together. We have learned that side effects of many medications are usually dosage related.

Before discarding the possibility of medication due to possible side effects, you should be reminded that to not give a child medication that he/she really needs to increase successful managing his/her behaviors or emotions is just as wrong as over-medicating the child with unnecessary medications or wrong dosage of medication. Perhaps you should look up the possible side effects of the common drugs that most of us wouldn't think twice about prior to taking—Aspirin, Tylenol or Ibuprofen. You will discover that even these drugs have a fairly long list of possible side effects and could be dangerous—perhaps even more dangerous than the medications recommended in your son or daughter's treatment. Please remember that just because the drug manufacturers and PDR list possible side effects to the medications, the vast majority of people taking medications do not experience these side effects when administered correctly and according to the doctor's prescription. All medications should be monitored closely by your child's physician and administered precisely as prescribed to reduce possible side effects.

PRINCIPAL MEDICATIONS used to treat anxiety disorders are anti-depressants, anti-anxiety medications, and medications known as beta-blockers. Although anti-depressants were developed to treat depression, they are also effective for anxiety disorders. The process is slow at first, taking about 2-3 weeks prior to noticing any changes; it usually takes about 4-6 weeks before symptoms start to fade. It is important to take these medications long enough to let them work.

Anti-depressant medications used to treat anxiety fall into 3 groups: SSRIs, Tricyclics, and MAOIs:

SSRIs (selective serotonin reuptake inhibitors) are some of the newest anti-depressants and considered some of the safest without addictive qualities. SSRIs alter the levels of the neurotransmitter serotonin in the brain, which, like other neurotransmitters, helps brain cells communicate with one another.

Prozac (Fluoxetine), Zoloft (Sertraline), Celexa (Citalopram), Paxil (Paroxetine), and Lexapro (Escitalopram) are some of the SSRIs commonly prescribed for panic disorder, OCD, PTSD, and various Phobias. A related medication that has some of the same qualities as SSRIs is called Effexor (Venlafaxine); Effexor has been found especially effective for treating General Anxiety Disorder.

SSRIs have fewer side effects than older antidepressants, but can produce slight nausea or jitters when people first start to take them. These symptoms can be significantly reduced by starting at a low dose and slowly increasing to the therapeutic dosage; and, generally any side effects usually cease within a few days.

Common side effects of SSRI medications include the following: dry mouth, nausea, headache, diarrhea, insomnia or trouble sleeping, sleepiness or over-sedation, nervousness, tiredness, constipation, sweating, abdominal pain, sexual response problems.

Tricyclics are older than SSRIs and work as well for treating anxiety symptoms, but have significantly more side effects that are more difficult to manage. Common side effects can include dizziness, drowsiness, dry mouth, and weight gain, which can be somewhat controlled by altering dosage or switching to a different tricyclic medication.

Tofranil (Imipramine) is prescribed for panic disorder and general anxiety disorder; Anafranil (Clomipramine) is sometimes used for treating OCD.

MAOIs (monoamine oxidase inhibitors) are among the oldest class of antidepressant medications and not frequently used since the more recent development of better medications with fewer side effects. People who are prescribed MAOIs need to go on a special diet since these medications interact with certain foods. MAOIs also interact with other medications, including some types of birth control pills, pain relievers (such as Advil, Motrin, or Tylenol), cold and allergy medications, and herbal supplements. Such interactions can be dangerous and cause serious increase in blood pressure. MAOIs and SSRIs cannot be taken together as well as the interaction can cause what is known as "serotonin syndrome" which can potentially be life threatening.

Nardil (Phenelzine), Parnate (Tranylcypromine), and Marplan (isocarboxazid) are MAOIs that have been used to treat panic disorder and social phobia.

Anti-Anxiety Medications are medications that fall into the medication class known as benzodiazepines. Benzodiazepines can be effective almost immediately, however, these medications may also become addictive, thus needing higher and higher doses to get the same effect; for this reason, these are usually prescribed for short periods of time.

Some people experience withdrawal symptoms if they stop taking benzodiazepines abruptly instead of tapering off, and anxiety can return once the medication is stopped. These potential problems have led physicians to shy away from these medications.

Klonopin (Clonazepam) is commonly used to treat social phobia and general anxiety disorder; Ativan (lorazepam) has been found helpful for panic disorder, and Xanax (Alprazolam) has been prescribed for both panic disorders and general anxiety disorder. Buspar (Buspirone) is slightly different than these other anti-anxiety medications and actually classed as an azapirone. Unlike benzodiazepines, Buspar must be taken consistently for at least 2-3 weeks to achieve any results. Possible side effects from Buspar include dizziness, headaches, and nausea.

Beta-Blockers are medications that are used to treat heart conditions; however, these medications have also been found helpful in the treatment of anxiety symptoms by preventing or better controlling the physical symptoms. Inderol (Propranolol) is a common beta-blocker prescribed to treat anxiety related symptoms.

IMPORTANCE OF ENVIRONMENTAL FACTORS

The influence of environmental factors appears to be very significant—especially in reinforcing or worsening the behaviors and characteristics of children. Some children have a very difficult time managing the transition from one activity to another. If the home environment is characterized by chaos, or lack of structure and consistency from one day to the next, the child may react with anxiety or insecurity. A predictable, fairly common routine from one day to the next is essential in creating a home environment that helps a child feel secure.

Most of us operate from a heavily stressed schedule, carrying our day-planners and palm pilot schedulers as well as cell phones that have become mobile computers that keep us on line with not only our office, but the world in general. Our typical tempo is excessive and we get very impatient if we experience traffic problems or highway construction that delays our arrival at our destination according to our planned arrival time. Children in this culture begin seeing this form of modeling from the adults in their lives quite early and as a result of significant modeling, they begin emulating this same behavior.

If a parent becomes stressed, nervous, apprehensive, or anxious over not meeting deadlines since they were "overbooked", they will model this form of response to stress; and, the child learns to respond in the same manner—thus learning anxiety perhaps innocently from the adult models they emulate.

Unfortunately, due to the busy schedules of their parents, some children only get parental attention when they have a "melt-down" and their emotions are displayed. These children suffer from what I have recently termed "PARENTAL ATTENTION DEFICIT DISORDER" or PADD. In such cases as PADD, the child begins learning to react with emotion to get his or her parent's attention, thus producing a pattern that can lead to the child getting "secondary gains" for the problem. As the emotional outbursts of anxiety, fears, panic, or phobias or other anxiety related symptoms are displayed, the child receives needed attention from the parental figure—thus the anxiety symptom is reinforced and becomes a strong motivator in accessing the desired parental attention.

HELPFUL INTERVENTONS FOR DEALING WITH MY ANXOUS CHILD

Most parents are anxious to learn more about helping their son or daughter who is struggling with anxiety symptoms. The following is a collection of ideas, gathered from various sources and many years experience, which might prove helpful to parents and teachers working with such children.

1. **Establish a structured environment with a very predictable routine:**
   - All children seem to do better with structure. Children who become anxious with the routine and expectations constantly changing will often express such emotions through increased anxiety, perhaps begin feeling insecure, experience insomnia or sleep difficulties, or some other form of emotional expression
   - The more predictable the routine and schedule, the better he/she will manage normal changes or events
   - Transitions from one activity to another can be challenging for many children; routines or schedules that form a consistent pattern seem to decrease the difficulty in managing the change in activities
   - When it is necessary to change the routine for some special event or crisis, prepare the child in advance by reassuring him/her of how the usual tasks will be handled
   - Verbally preparing the child about an impending change in routine, and giving them time to complete the current activity prior to the transition can reduce the stress or anxiety such a change poses for the child
   - School nights should have a consistent schedule that is kept with a specified time for homework, dinner, playtime, recreation or family time, bedtime, etc. that doesn't change from night to night or between caregivers
   - Morning routines should be similar with the same tasks expected each morning in preparation for school
   - A chart or written schedule of the routine will provide an excellent visual aid that can help the child stay on task and learn the routine

2. **Provide encouragement and remain positive and optimistic**

   - Be sure to reward or reinforce as many positive behaviors as those that are punished or disciplined; this helps to balance things and can help guard against damaging the child's self-esteem or inadvertently cause feelings of inadequacy or insecurity
   - Try to praise immediately any positive behaviors or successful performance; discipline for inappropriate behaviors can be delayed for better timing and the ability to process the misbehavior with the child
   - Look for ways to encourage and build up the child struggling with anxiety as such children typically are struggling with low self-esteem and feel his/her anxiety appears as weakness

- Teach the child to begin rewarding him/herself through self-talk (i.e. "You did very well remaining calm and not getting overly anxious...you are using those tricks well...and you are getting better each time you practice them"); this encourages the child to think more positively about him/herself and leads to optimistic thinking
- Give the child struggling with anxiety responsibilities which are within his/her capacity for success; this conveys to the child he/she is capable and helps to focus their mind on something other than the anxiety, worry, or issue causing fear
- Model for the child how you as an adult utilize coping skills to reduce the anxiety or stress that can suddenly appear on your schedule; try verbalizing your "self-talk" so the child can hear you as you work through the challenge productively and keep your worry, fear, and anxiety under control
- Be careful to model a positive and optimistic, hopeful attitude toward anxiety (i.e. help the child see that anxiety is a friend rather than a foe); anxiety helps us avoid dangerous or potentially harmful activities; neutralize the threat of anxiety by depicting it as one of many emotions we experience—it is just like others such as happiness, joy, anger, etc.

3. **Make necessary changes to environment in an effort to simplify it and neutralize the stressors or things that can lead to anxiety**

- Set up a separate room or part of a room as his/her special area for play or study; keep the décor simple and uncluttered; arrange a work table or desk facing a blank wall to avoid unnecessary distractions
- Reduce stimulation and possible distractions by turning off radio/ TV while performing tasks which require concentration (homework); multiple stimuli interferes with focusing on the primary task and can lead to anxiety when not successful
- Limit playmates to one at a time for the anxious child; by limiting the stimuli in the environment, he/she can experience more success socially
- Insure there is sufficient time for physical activity in daily schedule; it is important that children have a means of "venting" pinned up energy for this will help to reduce stress that can lead to anxiety
- Avoid over-stimulating or excessive schedules that often result when the child is participating in too many extra-curricular activities; encourage participating in one but avoid multiple or overlapping activities; avoid sports or activities that place unreasonably high emphasis on competition and winning
- While avoiding boredom, try to limit over-stimulation in schedule; routines, or home atmosphere
- Review goals and expectations of child to insure they are appropriate for age or normal developmental standards
- Surround the anxious child with "good role models" who are sensitive to

the child's needs and encourage him/her to try new things and provide appropriate peer support

4. Giving instructions or assigning tasks should be kept simple:

- Avoid giving complex or multiple tasks; keep things very simple and easy to understand; instructions should be short and clear
- Insure that the child understands the direction, task, or request by asking him/her to repeat it to you
- If necessary, repeat the task for the child in a calm positive manner— conveying a confidence that you know the child can accomplish this task or request
- Simplify or break down complex directions; instructions should be presented one at a time; avoid giving multiple commands
- Any list of rules should not be too long for the child to comprehend
- Posting the list of rules for a visual cue can be helpful
- Help the child feel comfortable in seeking assistance as many children will not ask for additional help or clarification
- Plan to give assistance longer for the child that struggles with anxiety; gradually reduce assistance as it becomes possible
- Maintain eye contact while giving verbal instructions; encourage the child to listen with his ears, eyes, and body—that helps to improve ability to focus on the task
- Be consistent with daily or repetitive activities/instructions
- Demonstrate slowly and carefully any new task or difficult assignment, showing the child the proper actions accompanied by short, clear, quiet, explanations; do not over-load the child's short-term memory; repeat the demonstration as often as necessary and until learned; be patient as the anxious child may take longer than expected to remember concepts
- Do one thing at a time; give the child one toy at a time to play with or assign one task at a time for him/her to accomplish

5. Provide appropriate supervision and practice limit setting:

- Place appropriate boundaries or limits on the child to help him/her make good decisions and be successful in their endeavors; the anxious child often lacks the ability to think through the consequences of an action prior to deciding to do it
- Remain calm while verbalizing the infraction of a rule or misbehavior; don't debate or argue with the child; never argue with the anxious child, it will only tend to escalate the frustration of both the child and the adult involved
- While it might be appropriate to administer the consequences immediately, it will often be more effective if you let the child know that consequences will be forthcoming but determined at a later time;

sometimes delaying the consequence is effective to deter further misbehavior as the child experiences what we call "therapeutic anxiety" while awaiting further action on his/her misbehavior; this form of anxiety is not harmful and should not be confused with anxiety in general; "therapeutic anxiety" will help the child think about his misbehavior and the consequences it brought to him/her—the ultimate goal of ALL DISCIPLINE is the get the child to think about his behavior and choices

· Discipline should be focused on learning rather than mere punishment; administer discipline without harshness but remain as neutral and non-reactive as possible

· Avoid any ridicule or criticism; remember the anxious child has difficulty staying in control—it is the nature of anxiety to lead a child to impulsive decision making and much patience is required in helping the child learn to slow down so he/she can learn appropriate problem solving

· Avoid publicly reminding the child of his problem; avoid correcting him in public when possible; discipline should be handled privately in most cases

· Learn to recognize warning signals that can help predict future problems; when they appear, quietly intervene, adjust the task, remove the child from the immediate environment, or redirect the child's focus in order to prevent anxiety from escalating

· Do not pity, indulge, be frightened by or manipulated by the anxious child; the anxious child needs to see your strength not weakness as an adult; by the adult taking charge, the child is relieved that things will be okay

· Do not give into secondary gains or manipulation that the anxious child may attempt in getting his/her own way; if the child has seen that his parents or other adults "react" whenever anxiety is displayed, this could lead to the child utilizing his/anxiety in a controlling or manipulative manner in an effort to get more attention or what he/she desires

6. **Try to enlarge your patience and ability to tolerate the various idiosyncrasies that most children who experience anxiety problems exhibit:**

· Accept the fact that the child may not at first be capable of managing his/her anxiety and the behaviors that accompany it—he/she can learn adaptive behaviors and coping skills with sufficient time, training, and support

· Don't personalize the child's anxiety or feel guilty that the child's anxiety is automatically a result of poor parenting; while the child may have seen it modeled with other family members and learned it as an inappropriate response to stress, many things can cause anxiety, and parents should avoid automatically claiming blame; remain positive and optimistic; the anxious child needs to see significant others in his life conveying hope that he/she can learn ways to deal with anxiety

· Practice the philosophy: "Problems are Opportunities" as you approach

106

or strategize handling the child's anxiety; most all problems are merely challenges that can be solved with the appropriate help and efforts

- Get support from others in handling the daily frustrations by talking with other parents or teachers; you will discover that as you share frustrations with others, this form of "venting" is therapeutic and seems to enlarge your patience as well as provide a supportive means of sharing ideas that have been helpful
- Try to remember that the anxious child is a unique person who needs help in learning appropriate expression of his emotions, rather than see him/her as abnormal, a problem, an embarrassment, or having a non-reversible disorder
- Expand your knowledge base regarding this condition through available resources (i.e. books, audio and video media, seminars, workshops, etc.)
- Each evening, take a moment to think about the day and to forgive the child for any possible transgressions; acknowledge that anxiety is not a condition the child wishes to possess; don't allow the stress of the extra measures required to support the anxious child to adversely affect your love for and relationship with the child
- Be sure to have "special times" with the child for recreation, fun, or relationship building times; such times will help to counter-balance the times of needing extra support when the child is displaying anxiety

7. Some helpful hints for the adults working with anxious children:

- Avoid falling into the trap of being endlessly negative: (i.e. "Stop...you are getting scared when there is nothing to be scared about...grow up....stop crying...there is nothing to be scared about...stop acting like a baby...!")
- Remember that under stress, people tend to regress to previous habits; re-directing the child who has regressed to expressing anxiety or fear is better than viciously confronting him/her
- Don't personalize the child's anxiety even if he/she verbally blames you—it's not about you so don't take it personally or get defensive and reactive
- Try hard to keep your emotions under control; try to appear "cool, calm and collected" despite feeling stressed; the child's anxiety will more quickly be reduced if he/she perceives the adults as in control and helpful to him rather than anxious and not knowing what to do to help
- Keep your voice calm; speak quietly and slowly as this approach can help to de-escalate the child and perhaps prevent the escalation that can end in a crisis or more anxiety
- Avoid using analogies—things must be kept simple and straight forward
- Don't lecture the anxious child; when intervening because of a misbehavior or display of anxiety, keep it simple and brief; anything longer than 5 minutes becomes a "lecture" to the child and he/she will

be apt to "turn you off" or discount the content of the discussion

· Do not make promises (implied or explicit) that you cannot/do not plan to fulfill
· Look diligently for positive behavior which you can reinforce; be sincere when praising the child as he/she will quickly discern any lack of sincerity
· Remember to make a distinction between the behavior you do not like and the child him/herself who you love (i.e. "I love you, but I don't like the way you are treating your sister..."); anxious children often misperceive disciplinary interventions from parents and teachers and this leads to increased anxiety if feeling unaccepted or unloved
· KNOW YOURSELF! Be aware of our own personal "hooks" or those things that might trigger anxiety or some other emotional response in you; if you struggle with anxiety as a parent, work on it so you can model optimism and hope in conquering it for your anxious son or daughter

8. Provide a MODEL for appropriate expression of ANXIETY

· James Dobson, Ph.D. has said that "more things are caught than taught" in child development; it is important that the adults around children provide a role model of what appropriate handling of stress or anxiety looks like; children generally learn to respond to situations in the same manner they see the adults in their lives responding to such things
· Relationship will probably be the most powerful tool an adult has with a child; a good relationship will have a positive influence in enabling both the parent and teacher to suggest alternative ways to handle stress or anxiety. As the child's relationship increases, he/she will want to please the adult and therefore be open to that adult's suggestions
· Without the foundation of a good relationship with the child, many parents and teachers resort to intimidation, threats, or fear as a means of forcing/imposing their will upon the child
· To create a good relationship with the child, the adult must be seen as:
    a. Fair—avoiding favorites, and not over-reacting
    b. Honest—always telling the truth, living up to promises made
    c. Caring—getting involved with the child's life, sharing self with child, becoming interested in the little things important to the child
    d. Right—demonstrating a sense of right vs. wrong
    e. Responsible—explaining rules, but being flexible; demonstrating a willingness to compromise when possible
    f. Dependable—keeping any promise made
    g. Respectful of others—mutual trust demonstrated for the other
        parent, co-workers, teacher, etc. (i.e. children can trust you since you trust others and others trust you)

9. Remember that all behaviors—both positive and negative—are valid and have meaning; anxiety needs to be understood, not scorned, ignored, or punished; understanding the behavior can eliminate the need to intervene or helps to plan appropriate interventions to correct or better alter the pattern

COMMON MYTHS THAT WORRY PARENTS

1. Anxiety problems are the result of poor parenting:
While poor parenting techniques can worsen or enlarge a child's problem with anxiety, it is not always the result of poor parenting. Some children are born with a tendency toward anxiety and thus will have less tolerance for things that might frighten or scare them. Such children might also have parents or significant others in their life that display anxiety when stressed or facing a challenging situation and thus the child's tendency toward this response is reinforced as it is modeled for them as the typical response in such situations.

2. Labeling a child with a diagnosis of Anxiety, Panic, OCD, or PTSD is harmful:
Labels are tools that help us in organizing and understanding concepts. In the case of properly diagnosing a child, then assigning that label to him/her could facilitate providing that child with the proper treatment and accommodations necessary for success. A diagnosis is far better than labels given to these children by their peers and even some teachers ("weird...weirdo... crazy... problem child... weakling... fragile..." etc.).

3. Children with anxiety problems usually always have ADHD, learning disabilities, or some other problem as well:
While the child experiencing anxiety may have other problems such as ADHD or learning disabilities, a problem with anxiety can and often does stand alone. Don't assume such a child's anxiety is multi-focused or caused by multiple things or conditions.

4. Medication should only be a last resort and only given when nothing else works:
While medication may be indicated to help reduce anxiety symptoms, it is not always indicated. When a child is exhibiting compensatory behaviors that appear to be symptoms of anxiety, it is often helpful to consider a small dosage of one of the anti-depressant medications. However, medication alone to treat the child with anxiety is never appropriate; other interventions including therapy, parental guidance and support, and environmental alterations are absolutely necessary even if the child is taking medication to help reduce his/her symptoms. It is most important that the

child learn better coping skills and gain understanding of the appropriate expression of this emotion rather than merely suppressing it.

To avoid giving a child medication when really necessary to treat the problem is neglectful! It would be just as bad to under-medicate as to over-medicate or use medication when it is not needed. Medication helps the child manage symptoms that are neurologically or chemically based while cognitive-behavioral therapy and environmental interventions help him/her develop coping skills for better managing this emotion.

The child's pediatrician or family physician should always be consulted whenever medication is recommended; in fact, coordination of the child's treatment with the pediatrician or family physician is highly recommended even when medication isn't part of his/her care.

5. **If I agree to use medication with my child, I can skip the therapy or other treatment suggested to treat his/her problems:**
While medication may help to reduce symptoms, it will be important that the child learn coping skills and better ways to deal with stressful situations. This is the purpose of therapy—to help the child replace previous habits with newly learned methods and coping skills. It is hoped that by applying his/her new learning and coping skills, the medication can be temporary and eventually discontinued. It is important that the physician who prescribed the medication take charge of the discontinuation rather than the parent or child doing this on their own.

6. **The only medication available for treating children with any problem seems to be Ritalin or one of the other drugs like Ritalin:**
While at an earlier time in history, Ritalin (methylphenidate hydrochloride) was probably the preferred if not the only medication that had been approved and therefore utilized in the treatment of children's hyperactivity, impulsivity, and related problems, drug companies have continued to work on discovering and developing better medications with significantly fewer side effects than Ritalin. Subsequent to the Ritalin era, additional mediations have been approved for treating children with a variety of symptoms. There has been a move toward the SSRI anti-depressant medications (Prozac, Paxil, Zoloft, Celexa, Lexapro, and others) due to their safety and ease in monitoring. Perhaps one of the best advantages of utilizing the anti-depressants rather than other medications is that dosing is usually once per day, they are not addictive, the benefits of the medication last longer into the day with few, if any side effects experienced.

7. **Physicians are too prone to prescribe medication without considering side effects and the severity of the child's problem:**
Most pediatricians and physicians are essentially not willing to prescribe any medications without a thorough evaluation of the child's condition and then will insist that the child see a psychologist, counselor, or therapist in addition to taking the

appropriate medication. When the medication is being prescribed, the physician will want to discuss such things as: (a) the child's age and weight, (b) the severity of the symptoms, (c) the specific target symptoms that will be treated by the medication, (d) whether problems such as learning disabilities, enuresis (bed-wetting), anxiety or depression need to be considered, (e) if a long-acting or short-acting medication would be more effective, (f) how often and when the medication should be taken, (g) possible side effects of the medication, (h) the child's feelings and attitude about taking medication, and of course, (I) the parent's feelings about their son or daughter taking medication.

8. I have heard that taking anti-depressant medication could increase the risk of my child having suicidal thoughts and therefore might increase the risk of suicide:

Unfortunately, there has been increased alarm about the possibility that taking anti-depressants can increase the risk of suicidal thoughts; however, there seems to be insufficient evidence to support such a notion. While some people that take anti-depressant medications have in fact committed suicide or made an attempt, this does not mean that the medication they were prescribed caused these thoughts or impulsive behaviors. One could utilize the same analogy about attending church, since some people who attend church have experienced suicidal thoughts or even completed suicide. Your doctor can explain that the medication is used to help re-establish the chemical balance within the body and really is not a "mind altering" drug.

9. Treating children with medication leads to drug dependency:

Research in drug addiction and dependency does not support the notion that children who are properly diagnosed and prescribed appropriate medications to help manage various symptoms such as anxiety later become addicts. What appears more predominant in clinical practice is the connection between children who were not treated with medication that could have been helpful and their subsequent drug usage and possible addiction. By the time the untreated child reaches middle school, his or her frustration is so high that it isn't unusual to find experimentation with alcohol, pot-smoking or other drug usage "to feel better." Properly diagnosed and treated children don't seem nearly as likely to experiment with drugs during middle and high school years. Some experts actually believe that appropriately administered mediation may help prevent children from developing more serious problems, and thus reduce the risk of such experimentation that is common among junior high or high school students.

10. Food allergies may cause behavioral changes in my child:

While some children appear more affected or show increased sensitivity to certain food products such as sugar, milk, nuts, chocolate, or preservatives and food dyes, scientific evidence does not give strong support for the role of food allergies or sensitivities causing various behavior problems. Obviously a reduction of sweets or foods containing excessive preservatives and dyes would be a good decision; however this should be done in the most inconspicuous way possible and not in a manner that could cause stigma to the child among his/her peers.

11. Medications will change my child's personality, will make him/her like a "zombie" or otherwise over emotional:

While in the past many children who were medicated for hyperactivity or attention problems were quite often over-medicated and therefore experienced several side effects such as these, recent changes in the manner in which doctors prescribe this medication has significantly lowered the risk of side effects. We have slowed down the whole prescribing process and start the child on the very smallest dose possible which generally causes no side effects. The doctor then slowly increases the medication (this process is called "titration") until the appropriate dosage is reached. Medication is used only to help the child better manage his behavior and reduce his/her propensity to over-react or have increased needless anxiety—not alter his thinking or emotional/behavioral state. The medication will not alter his emotional state or change his personality; it will only help him/her be able to exhibit the true personality which will be more positive and rewarding than the anxiety and associated behaviors that previously characterized him/her. The child's self-esteem is usually improved since he/she is getting far less negative feedback from the adults and finding peer relationships easier than before being on the medication.

12. Rather than use medications, using natural products such as herbs or natural foods and substances are safer:

Essentially, there is very little control over the herbal/natural food products in the USA. The FDA, a governmental agency that controls the production and usage of all medications, does not and will not obligate itself to also manage the herbal products. While there may be some products that could be helpful, we still don't know enough about these products and what they do within the body. The rigorous testing and standardization that FDA requires for all medications prior to approving them for the market is not done with the herbal/natural food product industry. We do not know how to dose them and what we do know about some of these products is still too limited to appropriately recommend their usage. Some parents claim that since these products are natural they are "safe." Most personnel working in such natural product stores have no formalized training and are recommending products that they claim are equivalent to medications prescribed by physicians who have had extensive medical training and practice. Many things come in natural forms that are toxic and can have extremely dangerous side effects especially when combined with other substances or medications. Arsenic comes in the natural form, but we know that it is poisonous and will cause death. Until further study and control of these products can be established, we discourage their usage unless specifically recommended or approved by your physician.

13. Taking medication will lower my child's self-esteem:

Taking medication may actually do just the opposite; a child constantly getting into trouble for not participating due to anxiety or feeling insecure very quickly begins experiencing poor self-esteem and generally withdraws from others. He/she begins to feel a lack of control for emotions or feelings, and very often gives up trying to gain better control. Once the child's anxiety levels are more controlled with the help of medication, he/she will feel less uncomfortable and be more willing to try new things, more willing to join peers in various social events, feel more normal or equal to peers rather than feeling "different" or "odd" as prior to gaining such control of their emotions and feelings.

14. Medications will cause growth suppression in children:
While some medications may cause a decrease in appetite, the pediatrician or physician prescribing the medication will monitor this possible side effect closely and make appropriate alterations in dosage, time of administration, or type of medication to minimize this risk.

15. Learning while under medication will not transfer when the child is no longer medicated:
Learning is essentially more possible for the child who is properly medicated since his emotional responses are more within his/her control. He/she can give focus to what is being taught as opposed to worrying about whatever is causing frustration, fear, or disruption in his/her life. What is learned will not be lost after the medication is no longer necessary.

Ask your doctor about any concerns or questions you might have regarding the use of medications and appropriate management of them. Knowledge is a powerful tool that helps reduce our concerns and clarifies misperceptions we may have because of things we have heard or read.

Endnotes

American Psychiatric Association: Diagnostic and Statistical Manual of Mental Disorders, Fourth Edition, Text Revision. Washington DC, American Psychiatric Association, 2000.

PARENT'S NOTATIONS FROM TEACHERS, COUNSELORS, AND THEIR CHILD'S DOCTOR

CPSIA information can be obtained at www.ICGtesting.com
Printed in the USA
LVOW091037030613

336666LV00004B/30/P